Victory Over Chaos

by Blaine Layne

Self Published.

All scripture quotations are taken from the King James Version (KJV) of the Bible.

Printed in the United States of America

ISBN - 9781792113413

VICTORY

Over

CHAOS

Victory Over Chaos

Enuma Elish, the Babylonian creation story, is a peculiar mythological story. Tiamat, a salt water dragon and goddess of chaos, mingles with a fresh water god named Abzu. This takes place in the heavens before the sky and ground are created.

After their children are created, then the children begin to have offspring as well. They become so wild, crazy, and loud that Abzu is unable to ever rest. He decides to kill all the offspring.

Ea, the grandson of Abzu and Tiamat, finds out the plan. He is the wisest of the pantheon. He slays Abzu and takes his crown. Tiamat declares war, and she creates an army of dragons and monsters.

Now afraid, they all seek a hero, including Ea. Marduk, the son of Ea, is called upon. Marduk agrees to fight, but he sets terms. He will become the ruler and king of the pantheon when he is victorious.

Marduk sets out clothed in gold armor. He carries a club, a bow with arrows, and lightning bolts. He shines like the sun, and he defeats the monsters and dragons. He is left to do one on one battle with Tiamat.

They ensue an intense and devastating battle. Finally, Marduk uses an evil wind down the throat of Tiamat. She is unable to close her mouth or swallow Marduk. He launches an arrow down her throat. The arrow splits her heart, and she is slain. Marduk then splits her body. He uses one half to form the ground, and he uses the other half to create the sky and firmament.

———

Now, those are some major family issues! I personally am not a fan of this story or Marduk. This has uncomfortable connections for me to bel and Babylon in the Bible. So, why? Why would I use this story?

When you look at this story as a battle that takes place within each of us, it takes on a more profound meaning. It is no longer a bizarre and ridiculous mythological creation story. It is relatable.

You are probably wondering, how? How in the world is this even remotely relatable?

How many of us have ever made plans? We have a vision of what should happen and how it should go. This is representation of the children. The problem is, chaos is always there by your side.

The plans DO NOT turn out how you imagined. What do we do now? We try to fix, salvage, or possibly erase what we created. What happens next? It backfires on us! We end up making situations worse, and suddenly we have allowed the chaos to create dragons and monsters we must kill. Some might call them inner demons.

This is where we need the hero within us to rise! We begin a brutal battle. If we can win, then this is where we defeat the chaos in our lives. We can set the terms. We can bend and mold it to create our reality! I like to call this, "Entropy Management".

Entropy Management

Entropy:

- thermodynamics: a measure of the unavailable energy in a closed thermodynamic system that is also usually considered to be a measure of the system's disorder, that is a property of the system's state, and that varies directly with any reversible change in heat in the system and inversely with the temperature of the system
- broadly: the degree of disorder or uncertainty in a system
- a process of degradation or running down or a trend to disorder (merriam-webster)

The process of entropy in science is very complex, but it can be simply explained as the state of order and structure to the movement of disorder or chaos. For example, a new building is constructed with a paved parking lot. If we leave it without any maintenance, we can come back in 3 years and see the degradation of the building: vines and plants have taken over, cracks have formed in the wall and parking lot, the building has become unstable.

For Christians, we believe this is the result of living in a fallen and corrupt world.

"Therefore, just as sin came into the world through one man, and death through sin, and so death spread to all men because all sinned." - Romans 5:12

Regardless of beliefs, science and faith conclude we live in a state of decline. Things seem to naturally fall apart around us when unattended to. We must create structure for our lives in all things, including health.

I was involved in a study in college. We were given a list, and we had to prioritize them in our life. Ninety percent of people listed personal health last. What people do not realize is health affects all your other priorities. You may not see the immediate repercussions, but over time, it will affect the two most important things in people's lives, family and jobs (money).

How do we organize and structure our health? What if I am not an organized person? First, if you are reading this book, you have already decided to prioritize health and keep it important in your life. That is the first step. Congratulations! Second, you make little decisions. Third, you make the little decisions more than once to create habits by repetitions. Fourth, you produce muscle memory for success.

This is no secret formula. It is the same formula to succeed or fail in anything. Though, I think having an awareness of the formula does produce better results. Why? Because our body likes comfort and laziness. Like I said, this is a battle against yourself. There are no microwave solutions. This book is not

here to help you find shortcuts, but it is here to help you build the mindset of a hero, warrior, and conqueror.

From the moment we wake up, we have a battle. Our first little decision and battle to win is a simple one. Wake up! How many times do I hit the snooze? Decide to NOT hit the snooze and win a battle. Decide to go to sleep a little earlier, rather than stare at your phone in bed for an hour. Little decisions produce huge victories over chaos.

In health, decide what you are going to eat for breakfast. Decide what you are NOT going to eat for breakfast. I have found I slip and fall when I have not decided prior to a moment. Suddenly, I am at work, it is time for lunch, and I don't have time to be healthy. I must settle, and I make a regretted decision for bad fast food.

We must create winning habits, and our bodies and minds are going to hate it…at first. Once our mind begins to create a dopamine reward system, then it will love it. (We will talk more about that in the following chapters.)

Entropy Management:

- The recognition of the importance of little decisions, which leads to protecting your future self from chaos.
- It is the ability to assess a situation in the moment and forecast potential chaos.
- An investment in your future self by organization and preparation.
- Taking time and energy now to save time and energy in the future.

Don't Miss the Mark

"The most important thing is to have a vision, and that you have a goal. Without that vision and without that goal, you are just drifting around and you will not end up anywhere. People do not become successful by accident….maybe the guy who found gold in California, but don't count on that." – Arnold Schwarzenegger

In the Bible, sin is translated as missing the mark. It is a reference to an archer aiming at a target and missing. According to the Bible, we have all missed the mark at some point in our lives. How do we know we missed?

The target and goal are outlined specifically for us in The Ten Commandments. The closer you look at the whole Bible, the more detailed the target becomes. When setting goals, we must provide an outlined and detailed vision to aim for. It's not enough to say, I am going to lose weight and get in shape. I will always ask, How?

It is called S.M.A.R.T. goals. This is something I teach kids every year in school.

- **Specific** – List a specific goal. For instance, I want to weigh 180lbs. You should also ask who, what, where, when, and why?
- **Measurable** – Measure out the goal and steps toward it. How much should you lose a week to get to 180lbs?
- **Attainable** – How am I going to do this and is it a realistic goal? For instance, going from 200lbs to 180lbs is achievable, but going from 200lbs to 180lbs in two weeks is not realistic. Also, you need to assess what tools are required to attain the goal. In this instance, it would be diet and exercise.
- **Relevant** – Is it worthwhile? Think about other goals you have, and how it will affect those goals. Will it increase productivity?

- **Time** – When will you accomplish your goal? Let's say 4 months, because that is when you are getting married. That means you need to lose 1.25 lbs per week.

Now, we have a mark to aim for. We have found our focus! Nothing is vague at this point.

How do you keep focus when it gets rough and you have to fight chaos of life? I think this is the hardest part for people. This is why we see people every New Year drop out of the gym after 3-6 weeks. The key is "Relevance" in your smart goals.

- How important is it to you?
- Do you want to do just enough to lie to yourself?
- Do you have a superficial goal?
- Are you strong enough mentally?

These are all hard and provoking questions. These are the questions you must ask to defeat your inner enemy. People with meaningful goals are the ones who conquer. They have value in what they are fighting for. Knowing you need to be healthy is never enough. One day, you will find the excuse you have subconsciously been looking for.

A doctor asks his male patient, "How would you feel about another man sleeping with your wife?"

The patient, confused and taking in the reality of the question, replies, "What?"

The doctor proceeds, "You just had a baby girl, right?"

"Yes", says the patient.

"Do you want another man to walk her down the isle on her wedding day?" asks the doctor.

"No!" The patient exclaims.

"That is exactly what is going to happen, unless you make some changes and listen to me," says the doctor.

This is a true testimony. This doctor knew exactly what to say to the individual to give him relevance and focus for healthier living. Health is an investment to those we love, as well as ourselves.

Don't Keep Up with the Kardashians

"If I don't feel confident about my body, I'm not going to sit at home and not do something about it. It's all about action and not being lazy." – Kim Kardashian

"You never regret a workout, just the workout you didn't make." – Khloe Kardashian

"I'm really proud of my curves, and I hope all you curvy girls out there are embracing yours, too. It's important to work out and be the best version of yourself that you can be, but never feel like you have to be the skinniest girl in the room to be the prettiest." – Kim Kardashian

I think these are some great words and quotes from the Kardashians. I don't think they are the greatest role models, and actions speak louder than words. On the other hand, I also understand they are in the spotlight, which means unending and ruthless criticism. They have intense pressure to keep a certain image, regardless of age and gravity.

Yes, they are curvy compared to the skinny models we see on the runway, but they are still not a natural look for women. Their look has money behind it. I don't think changing your body or having surgery to enhance yourself is a bad thing, but don't present that look as being achievable naturally. In fact, unaltered photos have shown how unnatural they can look at times.

As Kim said, "strive and be the best version of you." Set up ATTAINABLE and REALISTIC goals. When I was younger, I wanted to look big like Arnold and be shredded like Sly. I didn't realize the drug enhancement behind the look, or the extreme work and diet behind their figures. I thought going to the gym and lifting was the key.

The reality of that was very hard for me to digest. These guys were my heroes growing up. My Dad and I loved watching their movies together. I realized I had to change my goal for my image if I intended to stay natural. Hence, I found Steve Reeves; He was a natural bodybuilder and actor from the 1950s. Ironically, he inspired Arnold and Sly.

Let's talk about the tips and tricks used for film and photos. We all know that both men and women have plastic surgery for facial features and other asset alterations. We know they have professional makeup artist to shade and enhance facial features, cleavage, and abs. Of course, we also know they have photoshop. What about the actors and models who are legitimately in shape and look fantastic? We look at these people and swear they are photoshopped, but they are not. What is their secret?

The first guess for most people will be anabolic steroids. That may be a huge factor for some, but most of the time, the bodybuilders and models will incorporate something else. It is called dehydration and depletion.

Many have either been training for a show or a photoshoot. They have timed out their best physical condition. They do not get photos during their off season. They get photos when they hit their peak condition.

Based on their metabolism, they will time out their carbohydrates to almost zero the last week to get lean. Then, thirty-six or twenty-four hours before a show or photoshoot, they will completely dehydrate. After having almost zero carbohydrates, 24 hours before, they will finally eat something with a lot of carbohydrates. What does this do? This sounds crazy, right?

The Dehydration makes their skin look very tight and the muscles ripped. The carbohydrates twenty-four hours before will make the muscles bulge and not look flat from the hard diet. It can be very dangerous, but it is very effective for the perfect look.

These are the tips and tricks they do not discuss very openly. They do very unhealthy things to give a very healthy look. Having abs and muscles do not make people healthy. In fact, I personally know more skinny people with high metabolisms that are unhealthy.

So be careful who you follow and desire to look like. Set a realistic goal for you to look and feel great. Remember, this is a lifestyle and marathon, not a sprint.

Get Dope!

We are not talking about marijuana, which reverts IQ points and creates an altered reward system. Although, the addiction to marijuana may come from this neurotransmitter. We are talking about dopamine, and more importantly, the dopamine reward system.

"Dopamine is both a neurotransmitter and a neurohormone produced in multiple areas of the brain. As a hormone it is often associated with pleasant experiences. Receiving an unexpected reward may cause your heart to speed up and increase your alertness due to the sudden release of dopamine." (alleydog.com)

Basically, this means it is the Paul Revere of pleasure. It signals and screams, "This feels good! Do it again!" This rises the question, how can exercise create and send dopamine, when you are punishing yourself physically and creating pain?

This is where endorphins come into play. Endorphins are the chemicals released to counteract the perception of pain and trigger positive feelings. A lot of times it is compared to the same effect as morphine. You feel good regardless of the pain and stress you have. In fact, you feel better than before you began to cause pain. This is why exercise is known to fight depression and increase self-confidence. I believe people who exercise create the psychology to conquer and battle everyday chaos, even laugh at it. They have developed a positivity under stressful conditions.

After experiencing and creating this process, next time you think about the gym, Paul Revere will send signals reminding you of how great you feel mentally after a workout. This is the reason people become addicted to coming to the gym.

Finally, let's talk about the reward system, which is connected to the dopamine as well. This is also the key to staying motivated and fighting the lie to yourself. We talked about S.M.A.R.T. goals earlier, and how setting these goals keep focus, especially when you have created high value for it. Detailed steps in the goal is very important. Each time you defeat a small or detailed goal, you begin to feel like a winner and a champion. Paul Revere comes and says, "Keep going. You are doing great!"

For example, even drinking 8-10 glasses of water in a day is a great achievement. It's a VICTORY! It is like a sports season. You want to win a game, and when you do win, you celebrate. Remember though, it is just one game, and you must win enough games to make yourself eligible for the championship.

Some of you may ask, "Blaine, what happens when I lose, and I have a bad day? What happens when it is no longer worth the fight?" That's a great question.

"I never saw a wild thing sorry for itself. A small bird will drop frozen dead from a bough without ever having felt sorry for itself." – D.H. Lawrence

Many of you may recognize this poem from the 1997 G.I. Jane movie, but it was written way before then. I think this poem is so intuitive with humans. Humans seem to have self-pity and loathing above all other creatures. Wild creatures seem to deal with chaos and circumstances better in the moment than humans. You might say, that is because they cannot look ahead to the future to prepare. I disagree with that, because they prepare for the winter.

I think there is a lot we can take from this two-sentence poem. My dad seems to do well with this. I have seen him come home, after a fourteen-hour work day in a foundry, and work on the yard, house, or cars. In fact, I finally asked him one day.

"Dad, how do you work all those hours in the foundry, come home and work more? It makes me tired thinking about it."

He replied, "That's it."

"That's what?" I asked.

"You think about it. If I thought about it, I wouldn't do it. It's something I know must be done, whether I feel like it or not. Don't think about it, just do it."

This has greatly impacted my life. My dad is currently in his sixties and still has the same work ethic and relentlessness. My mother is right up there too. My parents have challenged my mindset. If they can do it, why can't I? I have no excuses. That is the bottom line. Influences and perspectives shape our to mindset to battle.

Unfortunately, not all of us, have had these types of influences. Is depression linked to environmental factors? This is an ongoing argument and study of environment vs. genes. Studies do reveal environment is a larger impact than genes. Some have 60% environment factor and 40% genetic factor, but even the 40% is affected by the environment.

I personally do believe that environment is the biggest factor, but there are definitely genetic factors for people, especially those with chemical imbalances. One of those is serotonin. Serotonin is also a neurotransmitter like dopamine. Its function is to regulate your mood. It keeps things in balance, and a deficiency can lead to depression.

I believe depression and anxiety is one of the hardest obstacles for people to overcome. Exercise is one of the most successful ways to overcome it. Dopamine is the cause for reward and motivation, but how can you reprogram your mind if you have no motivation to begin with? Unfortunately, not everyone will have success in this. That's the cold and dreadful truth.

Once again, people who have success, they find the value for what they are fighting for. As a person of faith, I believe everyone has an infinite worth and value, even if they don't believe it themselves. A challenging verse I love is Matthew 6:34.

"So don't worry about tomorrow, for tomorrow will bring its own worries. Today's trouble is enough for today."

Wait. Are you saying we shouldn't plan ahead with entropy management? No. this verse is not saying, "don't plan ahead and take care of yourself." It is saying, "don't let chaos you can't control in the future, cause you to stress and worry today. Take care of the chaos today that you can battle and take care of."

Iron Sharpens Iron

"And Ishbi-benob, one of the descendants of the giants, whose spear weighed three hundred shekels of bronze, and who was armed with a new sword, thought to kill David." (2 Samuel 21:16, ESV)

This is the perfect example of having friends, family, spouses, and warriors to help you when you are in a weak state. David became infamous for killing the giant Goliath. He became known as "The Giant Killer". Ironically, nobody ever mentions the time he was almost killed by a giant smaller than Goliath.

In the midst of battle, David falls and Ishbi-benob, the giant, is about to kill David. It was his nephew and warrior, Abishai, who came to his aid and helped him when he had fallen.

"But Abishai the son of Zeruiah came to his aid and attacked the Philistine and killed him." (2 Samuel 21:17, ESV)

David was an extraordinary leader. He always set the example and standard. His men followed in his footsteps and took out giants when the known "Giant Killer" was unable to.

**"And there was again war at Gath, where there was a man of great stature, who had six fingers on each hand, and six toes on each foot, twenty-four in number, and he also was descended from the giants. And when he taunted Israel, Jonathan the son of Shimei, David's brother, struck him down."
(2 Samuel 21:20-21)**

We all need those warriors in our lives: friends, family, spouses. They are the ones to help us fight the chaos. Their strength can bring balance and rest when we need it.

I can tell you one important thing. If it wasn't for the support of my beloved wife, I could not do what I do. She stands by and encourages me 24/7. She helps me cook and prepare meals for our eating lifestyle, not diet.

She is not mad or jealous when I go to the gym. I am not mad or jealous when she goes to the gym. Believe it or not, this is something I hear quite a bit from men and women. It is such a blessing that I have her support.

I can also say this about my parents. They do not always agree with me, but they have always supported me, as long as I am not being self-destructive.

Next, it's my friends and lifting partners in the gym, like Derek, the COO of Victory Over Chaos, who push me to my limits to become my best. It's my teachers and mentors, who have taken time to talk and pour wisdom into me. I am not saying you cannot fight the battle by yourself, but it is so much easier when you have an army standing beside you.

Be Independent!

This may seem completely contradictory to the last chapter. It is preferable to have support and can be very vital to push you to the next level. Sometimes, we just do not have that luxury. This is another quality of being successful at your goals. At the end of the day, YOU must be the one to accomplish them.

There have been many times people have committed to helping me. When the time comes, they are nowhere to be found. If you wait on other people to accomplish your goals, then they will never happen.

Also, what about the people who are not supportive or understand your goals? Be careful who you tell your dreams to. One wrong conversation can murder your dreams and motivation. They will tell why you cannot do something, instead of telling how to overcome the "cannot". Problems to a goal are great to be presented and acknowledged, but a solution needs to follow.

Be Stubborn!

You should be stubborn about your goals too. I remember hearing so much negativity about my health before I got married. People were anticipating me to give up. Several people said, "All this health stuff and lifting you do will end after you get married. You enjoy it while you can." I remember my fight or flight kicking in. I felt challenged, and I didn't quit.

Next, I remember when I had kids. People said, "You won't have time to lift anymore." Once again, I didn't quit. Last, I started working two jobs and working 65 or 70 hours a week. Of course, somebody said, "I guess you won't have time to lift." Now, I am still working 65 or 70 hours a week, training 5 or 6 days a week, and I am starting the Victory Over Chaos brand.

You should refuse to let other people decide and design your goals. That does not mean you shouldn't listen to wisdom but block out "naysayers" who do not provide solutions.

Remove Die out of Diet!

It is true that a high percentage of your physique is contributed to your eating lifestyle. I have seen some place it at 80%, training at 10%, and genetics at 10%. I personally would range it around: diet 50%, training 30%, and genetics 20%. Regardless, it shows how important a diet or eating lifestyle can be.

Mentally and physically, I believe this is the hardest part of becoming healthy. Health is not all about outward appearance. We seem to focus and decide if someone is healthy by their appearance. I know more slim people with high metabolisms who are way unhealthier. When it comes to overall health, I DO place diet at 80%.

Let's be honest, sticking to a year around diet is probably not a realistic goal. I hate the terms diet and cheat. It should be lifestyle and reward. In my Road to Health packet, it is not my goal to get people to make 100% healthy choices. It is my goal to get people to make 50% healthier choices. This is a huge increase when you go from 0% healthy choices.

We are human, and we should be able to experience and enjoy life. I want a person who has worked very hard to go out on date and eat some cheesecake with their spouse or loved one. They have earned it. It is a reward!

It becomes cheating when people are eating bad every meal and not training themselves mentally or physically. They are not only cheating themselves, but time everybody has with them.

Less Talky. More Lifty.

"Focus!" – Dwayne "The Rock" Johnson

Many of us have seen the videos of The Rock screaming this during his workouts. Derek and I scream this at each other semi-joking during ours. Remember, chaos is everywhere, including the gym. All it takes is one greeting to lose your focus, pump, and motivation. Here are a few tips to prevent this.

1. Put your phone up. It is so tempting to look at texts, emails, and social media between sets. Although, I do connect my phone to my fit bit in case Mary needs to contact me for emergencies.
2. Wear headphones. This is a subtle way to let people know you are focused. There have been times my headphones are not charged, but I wear them anyway. This also provides the opportunity to give a

greeting with a nod or wave without having to stop working out.

3. Beware of caffeine and preworkout. I always take some form of caffeine, but the energy may cause you to talk more, if you do not find your muscle to mind connection.

4. Find a good workout partner. How do I find that? It's nice if you have a friend who likes to go with you occasionally, but usually they are going because they care about you and not the training. This can become a distraction too. I would say train hard and be consistent. You will eventually meet somebody at the gym with the same work ethic as you. My current training partners, Derek and Ace, have that tenacity to work hard themselves, which keeps me from slacking too.

5. Get in the zone. During the warm up, you should try to find the muscle to mind connection. You begin by lifting light weight to get blood flow and concentrating on contracting the desired

muscle. This will create a tunnel vision, and you become less aware of everybody else around you.

6. Don't compare. Form is always more important than weight. I can immediately tell if a beginner comes to the gym, and they feel uncomfortable. Many times, they will go and pick up the heaviest weight possible and sling it around. There is no form or focus. They just sling it! They could hurt themselves very quick. The gym can be very awkward and intimidating if you are new. There is so much equipment, and nothing is the same. Plus, the members can come across as intimidating. I am more inspired by someone stepping out of their comfort zone and making a change at the gym, than the guy curling a 100lbs with one arm. Don't compare and get distracted by other members. Do your thing at your level. Be proud that you are there!

Stay Hungry.

I hope everyone reaches their goals in health and life, but then there is always the lost feeling after you accomplish a goal. I feel like that every time I finish a show on Netflix. What do I watch now?

There is also the feeling of accomplishment to the extreme. "I have reached my goal. I guess there is nothing else left to do." We need to celebrate accomplishments, but we don't need to become idle. This can lead to reverting goals. Sometimes challenging yourself on an accomplished goal is good. For instance, "I lost 10lbs. Now, I am going to try and lose 5 more lbs."

Maybe, you just need to turn your attention to an entirely different goal. Whatever it is, don't stop moving forward and setting goals. We all have the ability to become winners, but only a few have the capability to program their mind to be heroes over chaos.

This book is about the mindset to Victory. That's where goals start and end! Like I said, I hope you reach your goal, but I also hope you fall a few times before getting there. If you are strong enough, you will learn from it and stay hungry. I hope your "fight" kicks in, when you feel the desire to take flight. I hope you all are content with your accomplishments, but never satisfied. Progress! Progress! Progress!

Victory Already Won!

We have been discussing how to overcome everyday chaos here on Earth, but we have already received victory eternally, if we will accept it. This victory was won with somebody else's blood, sweat, and tears. He loves you, and so do I. May God bless you, and I hope you let Jesus know that you believe in Him, and you acknowledge that He died to cleanse our sin. He will change and transform your life and mindset for the best.

Thank you all, and don't forget to check out our websites: blainelayne.com and vchealth.com!